Dedication

To all the children who read this book, may you become Super-Sleepers and choose to use Sleep Magic to discover your mighty SuperPowers to grow big and strong, bounce back fast when you're feeling ill, embrace learning with joy, and have the courage to make your dreams come true. Remember to treasure the wonderful gift of Sleep Magic every day to help nurture your talents and support all the amazing things you want to do.
Happy adventures and sweet dreams!

Doctor Bedtime's
Sleep Magic

KID APPROVED

Superpowers for Super-Sleepers

Written by

Roger Washington, MD and Scarlet Nickhol, MPP, MBA

Illustrated by

Stacy Hummel

For the

SLEEP TO LIVE WELL FOUNDATION

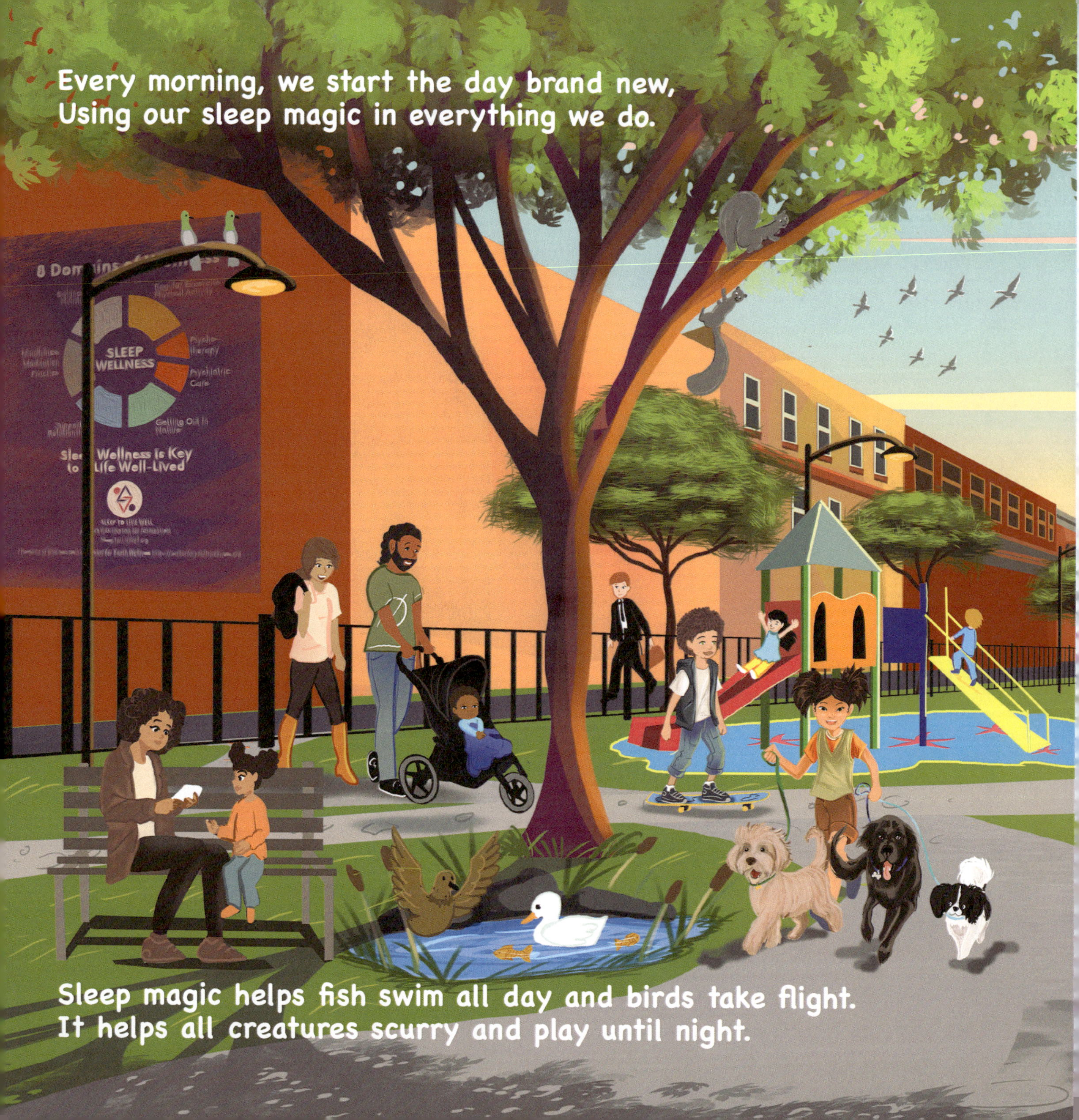

Every morning, we start the day brand new,
Using our sleep magic in everything we do.

Sleep magic helps fish swim all day and birds take flight.
It helps all creatures scurry and play until night.

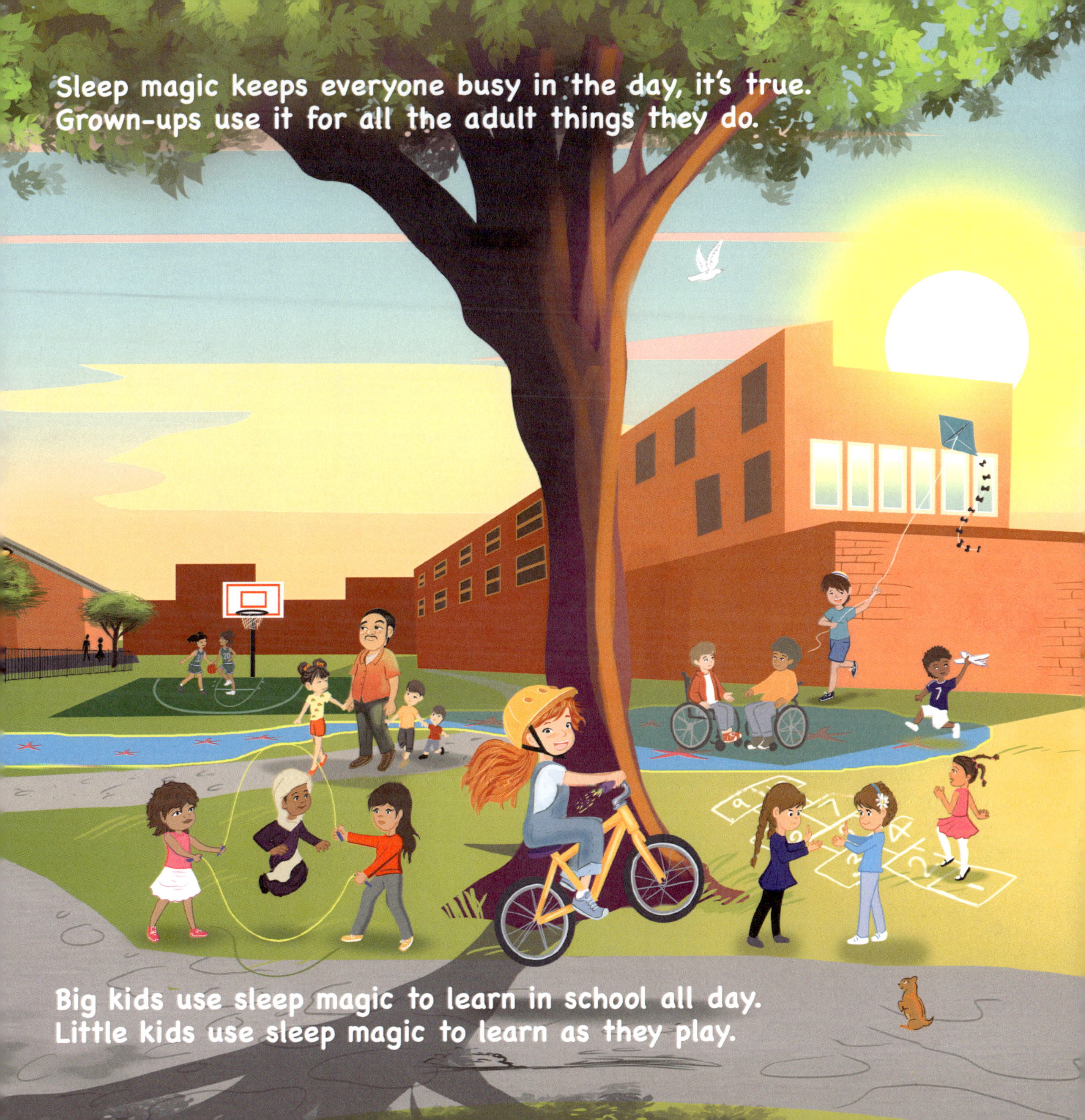

Sleep magic keeps everyone busy in the day, it's true.
Grown-ups use it for all the adult things they do.

Big kids use sleep magic to learn in school all day.
Little kids use sleep magic to learn as they play.

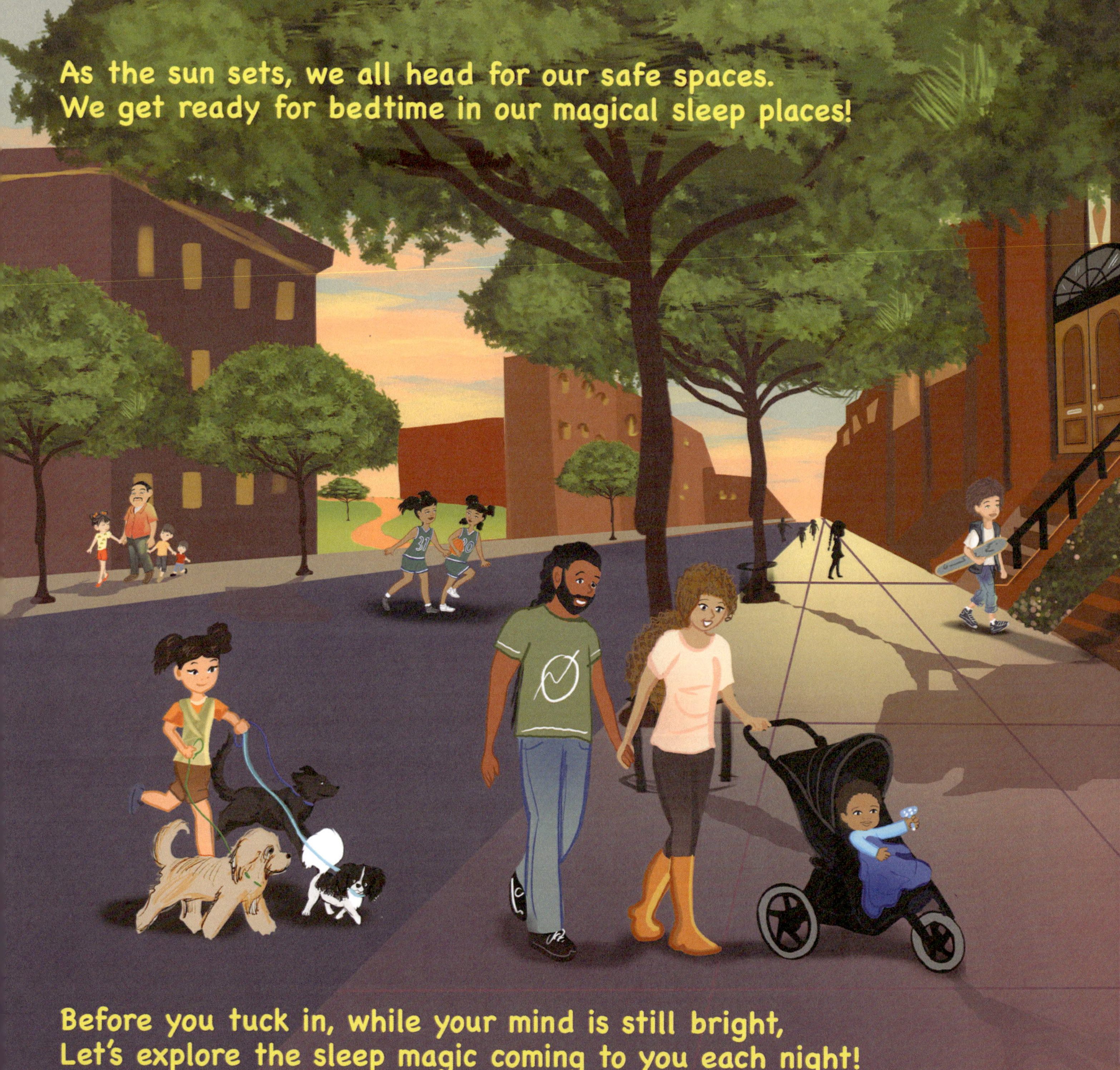

As the sun sets, we all head for our safe spaces.
We get ready for bedtime in our magical sleep places!

Before you tuck in, while your mind is still bright,
Let's explore the sleep magic coming to you each night!

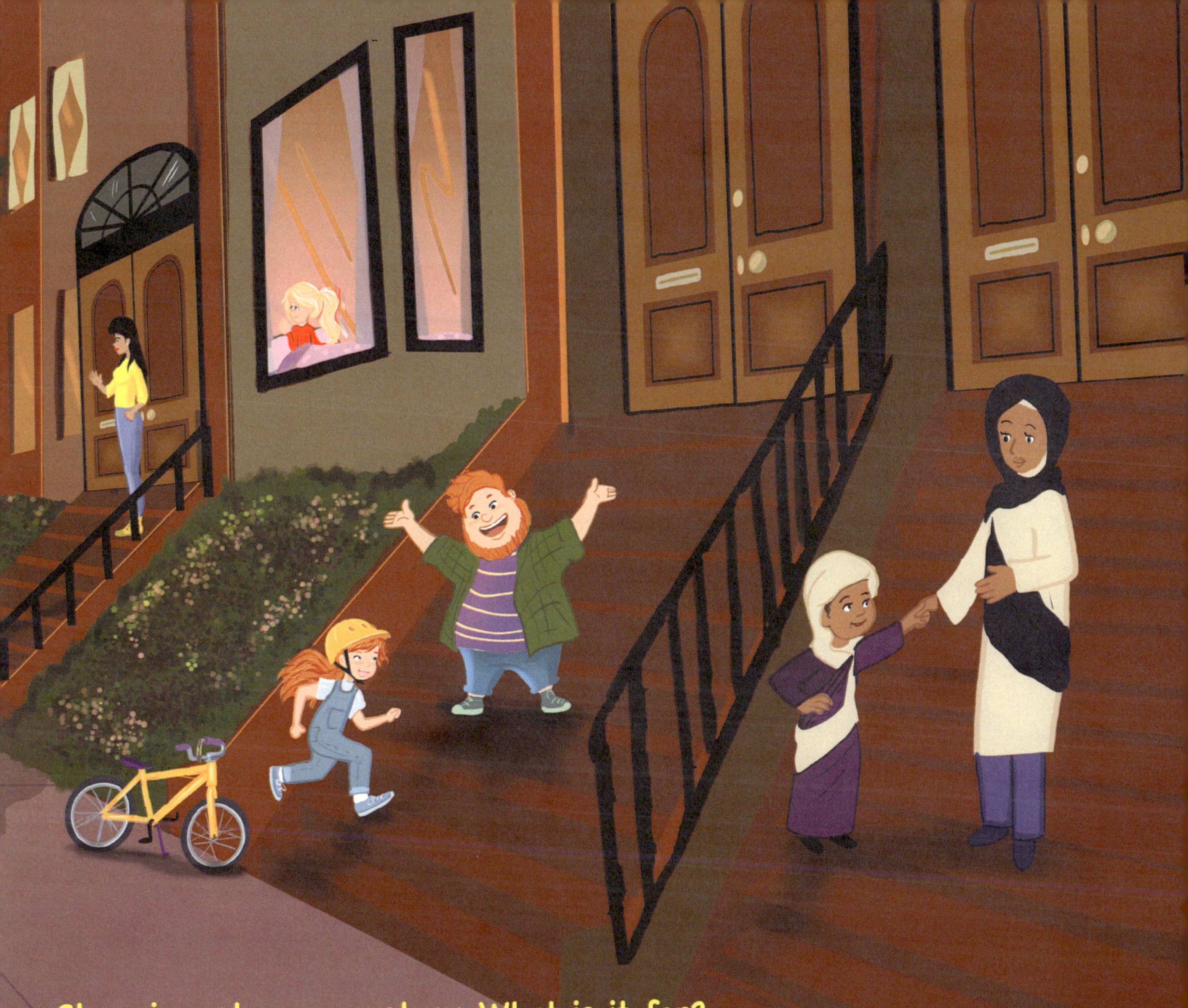

Sleep is a strange mystery. What is it for?
It gives you special SuperPowers. And it's time to get more!

Let's go to the places where sleep magic is found.
Where creatures get SuperPowers by sleeping safe and sound.

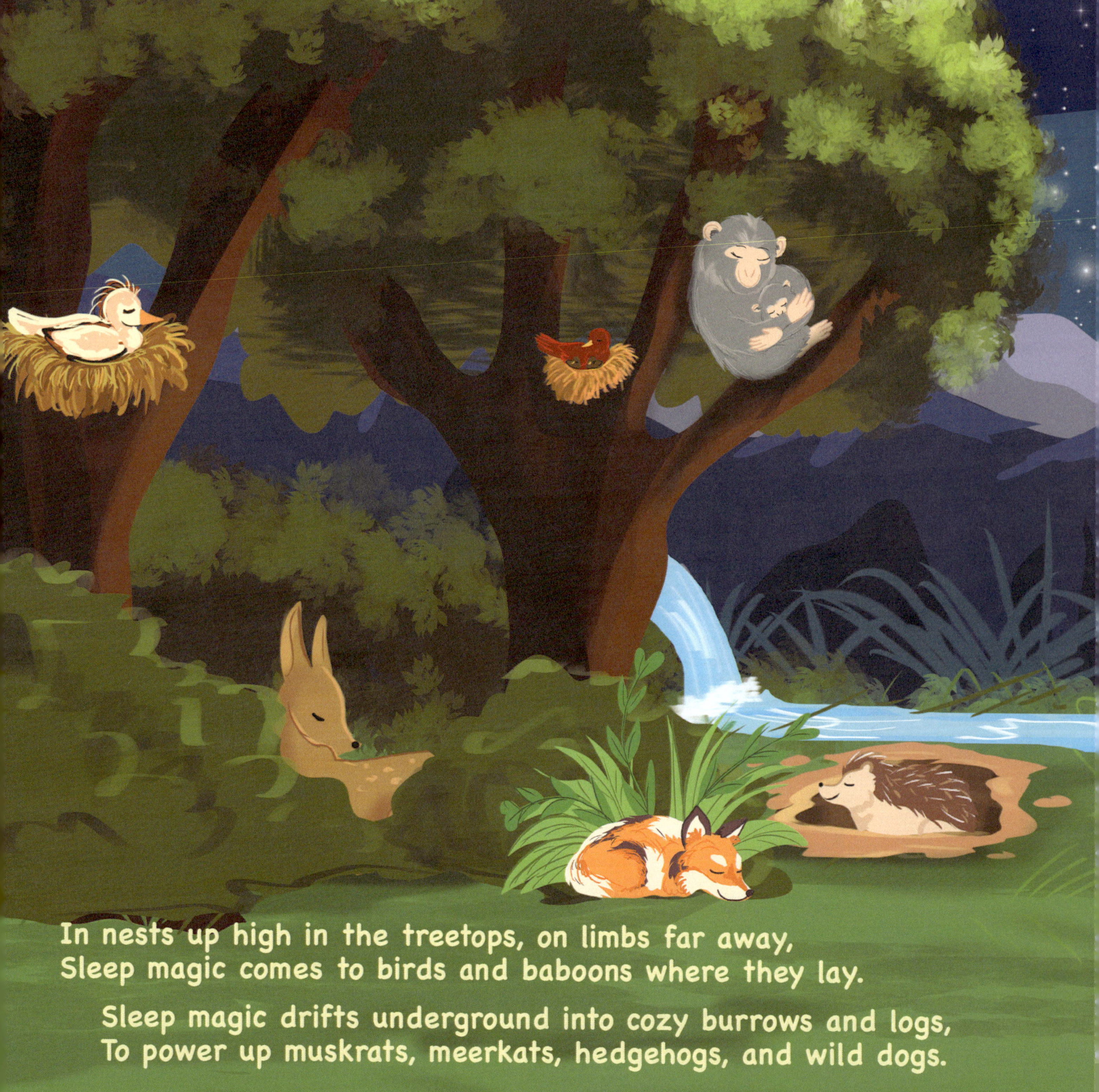

In nests up high in the treetops, on limbs far away,
Sleep magic comes to birds and baboons where they lay.

Sleep magic drifts underground into cozy burrows and logs,
To power up muskrats, meerkats, hedgehogs, and wild dogs.

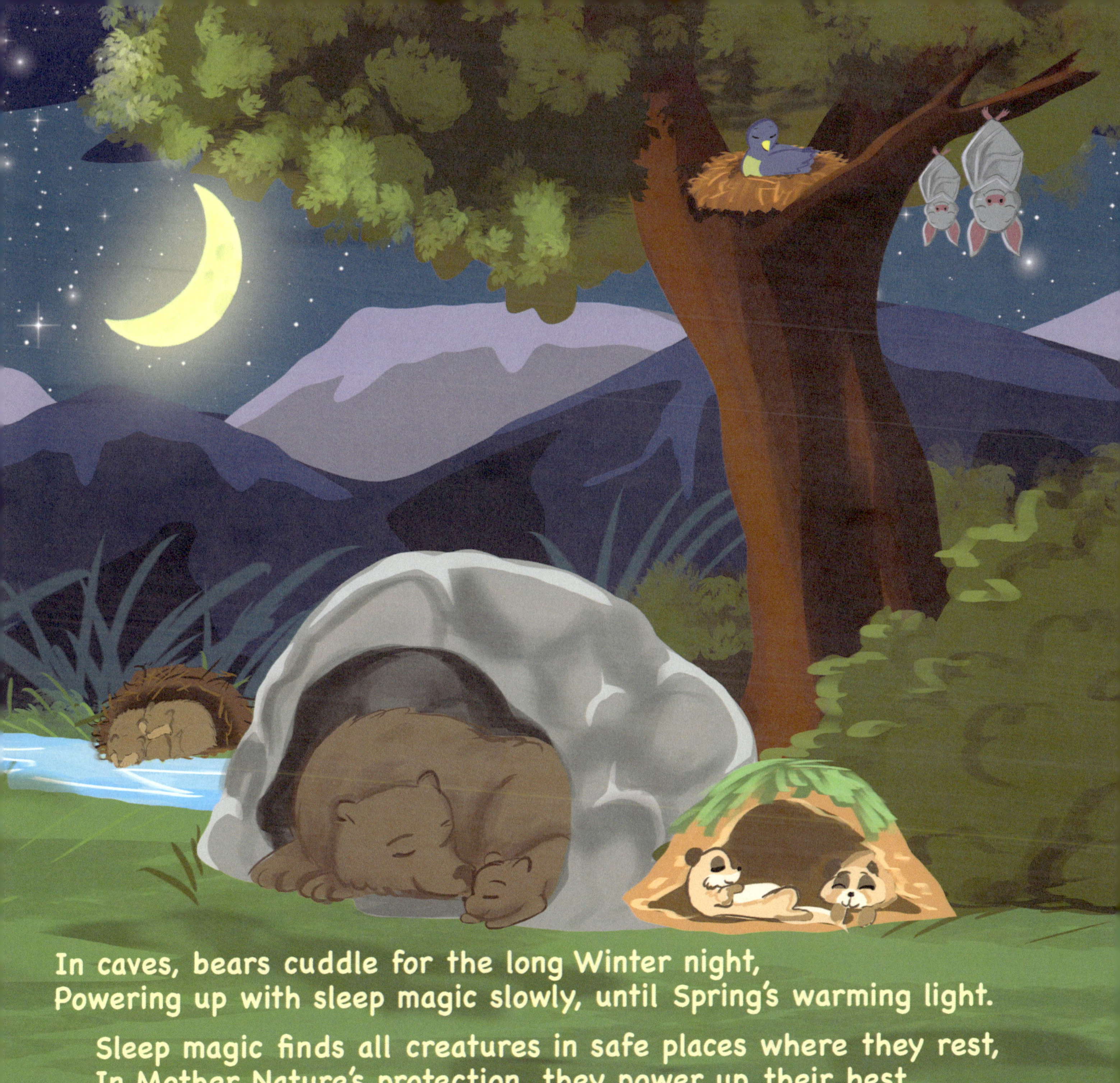

In caves, bears cuddle for the long Winter night,
Powering up with sleep magic slowly, until Spring's warming light.

Sleep magic finds all creatures in safe places where they rest,
In Mother Nature's protection, they power up their best.

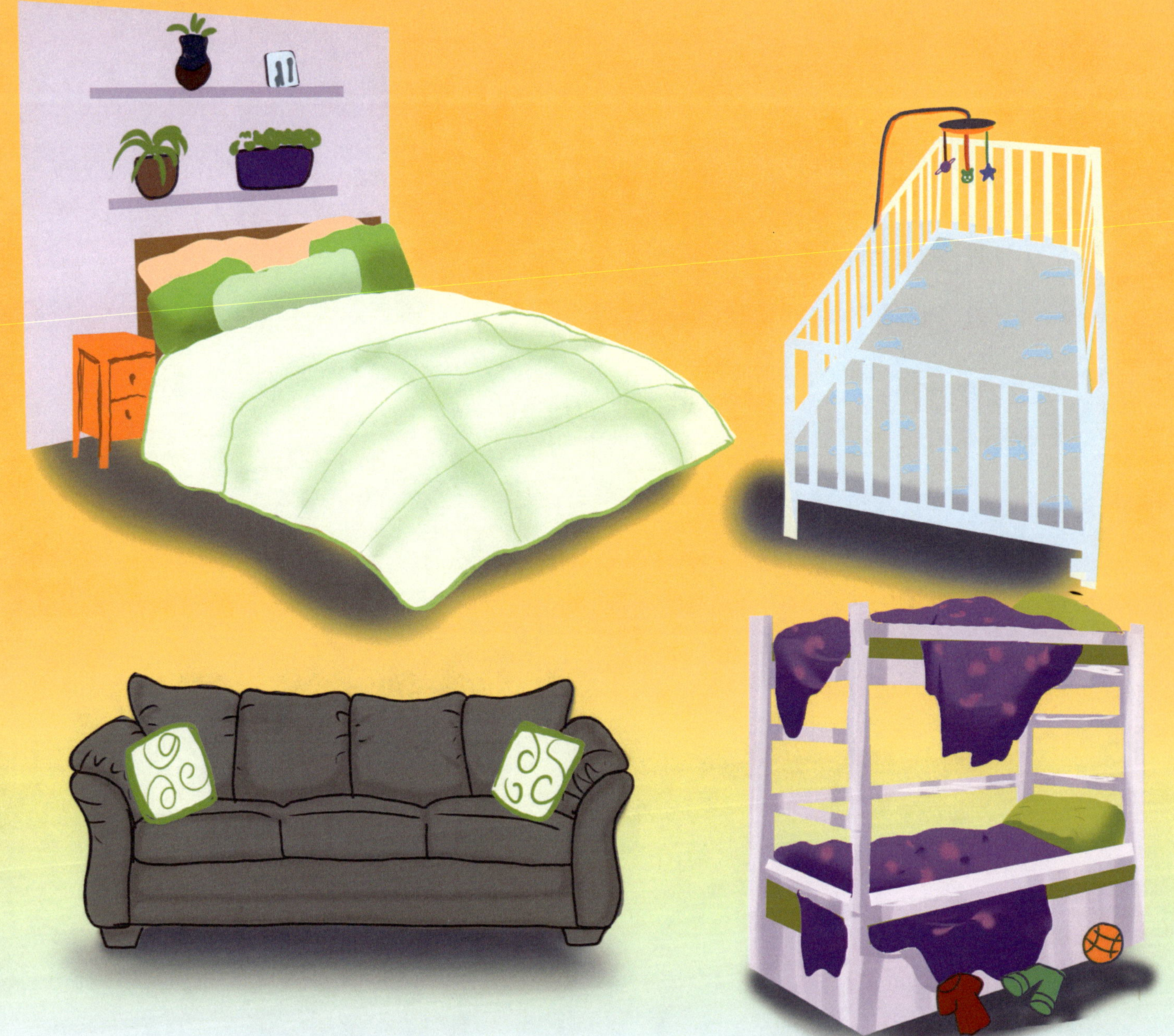

Where does sleep magic find you? When do you power up best?
In your safe space at bedtime, when you're ready to rest!

Beds made with pillows and blankets, sometimes with toys,
Starts the sleep magic flowing to all girls and boys.

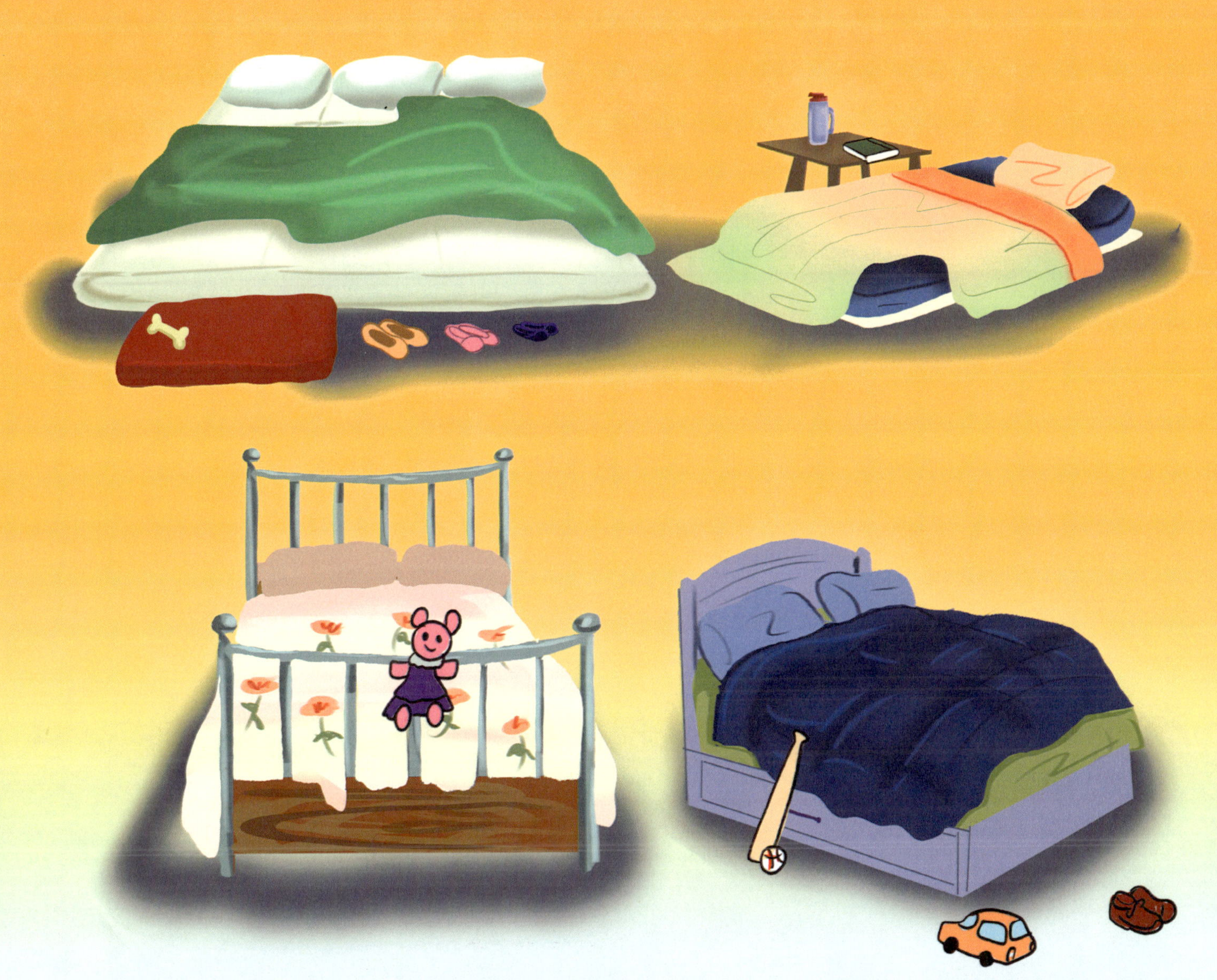

What about mommies, daddies, and teachers, too?
Where do they go for sleep magic when the day is through?

Parents and adults choose beds of all kinds,
And sleep magic comes to every safe space they find.

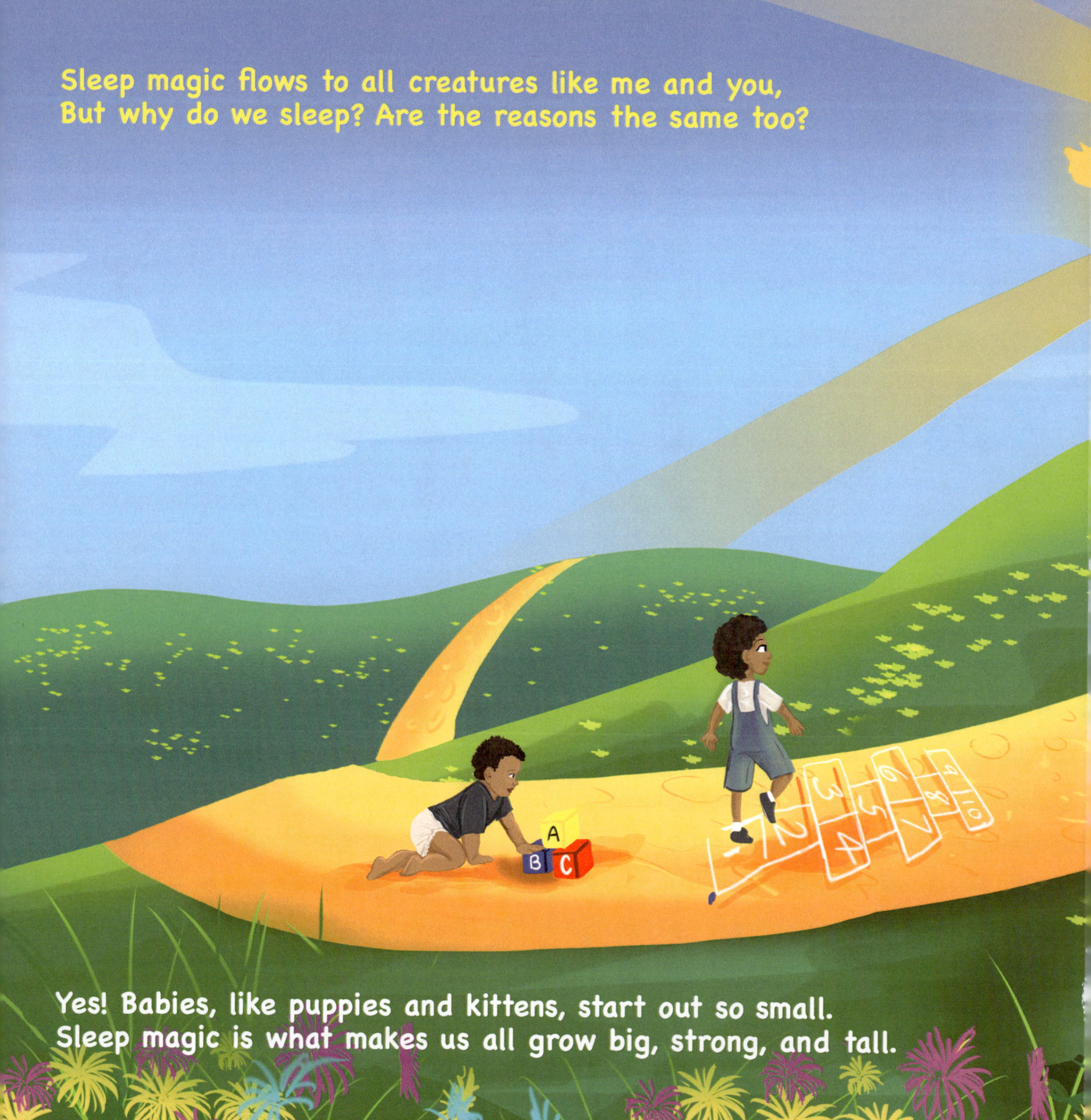

Sleep magic flows to all creatures like me and you,
But why do we sleep? Are the reasons the same too?

Yes! Babies, like puppies and kittens, start out so small.
Sleep magic is what makes us all grow big, strong, and tall.

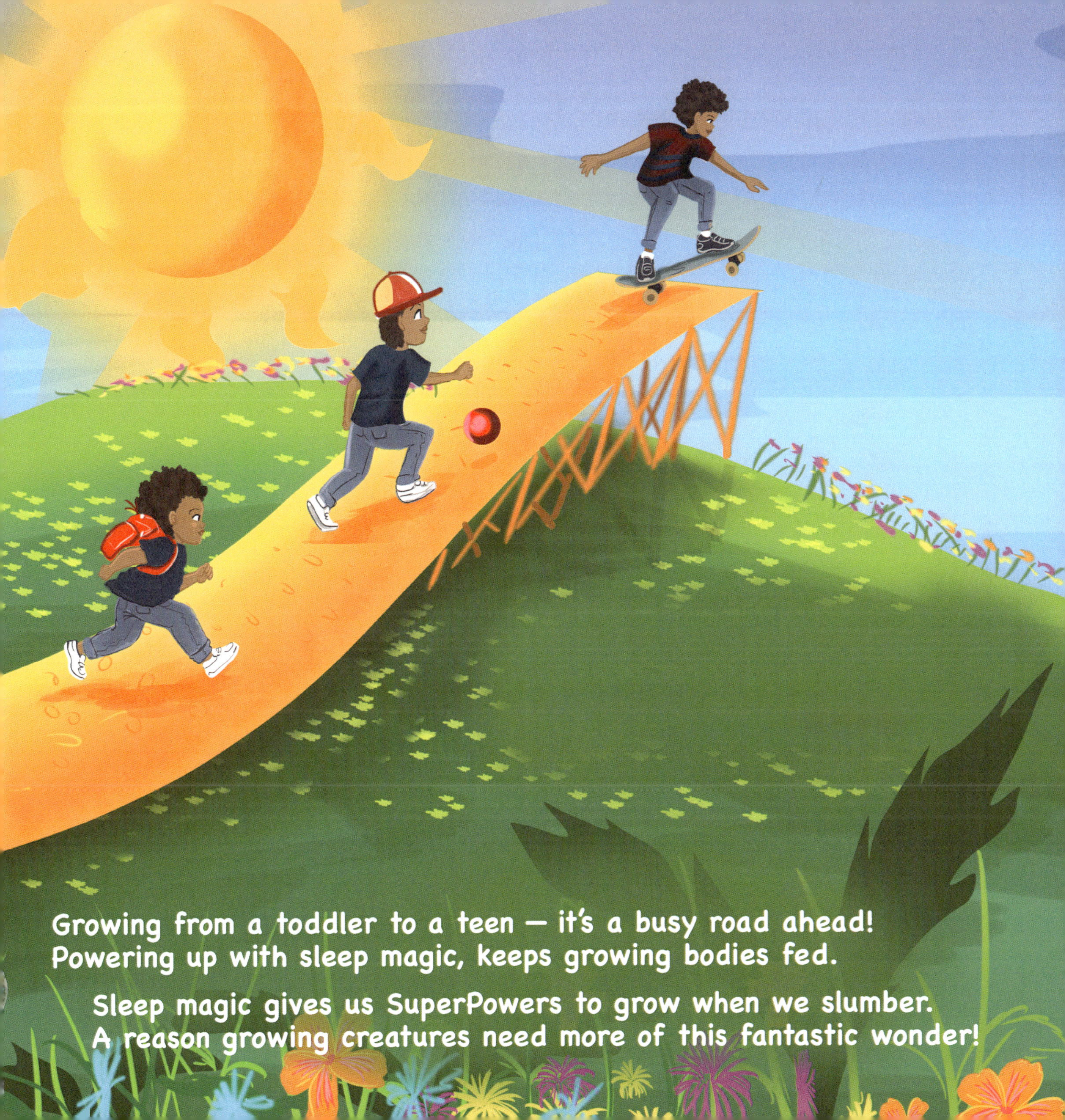

Growing from a toddler to a teen — it's a busy road ahead!
Powering up with sleep magic, keeps growing bodies fed.

Sleep magic gives us SuperPowers to grow when we slumber.
A reason growing creatures need more of this fantastic wonder!

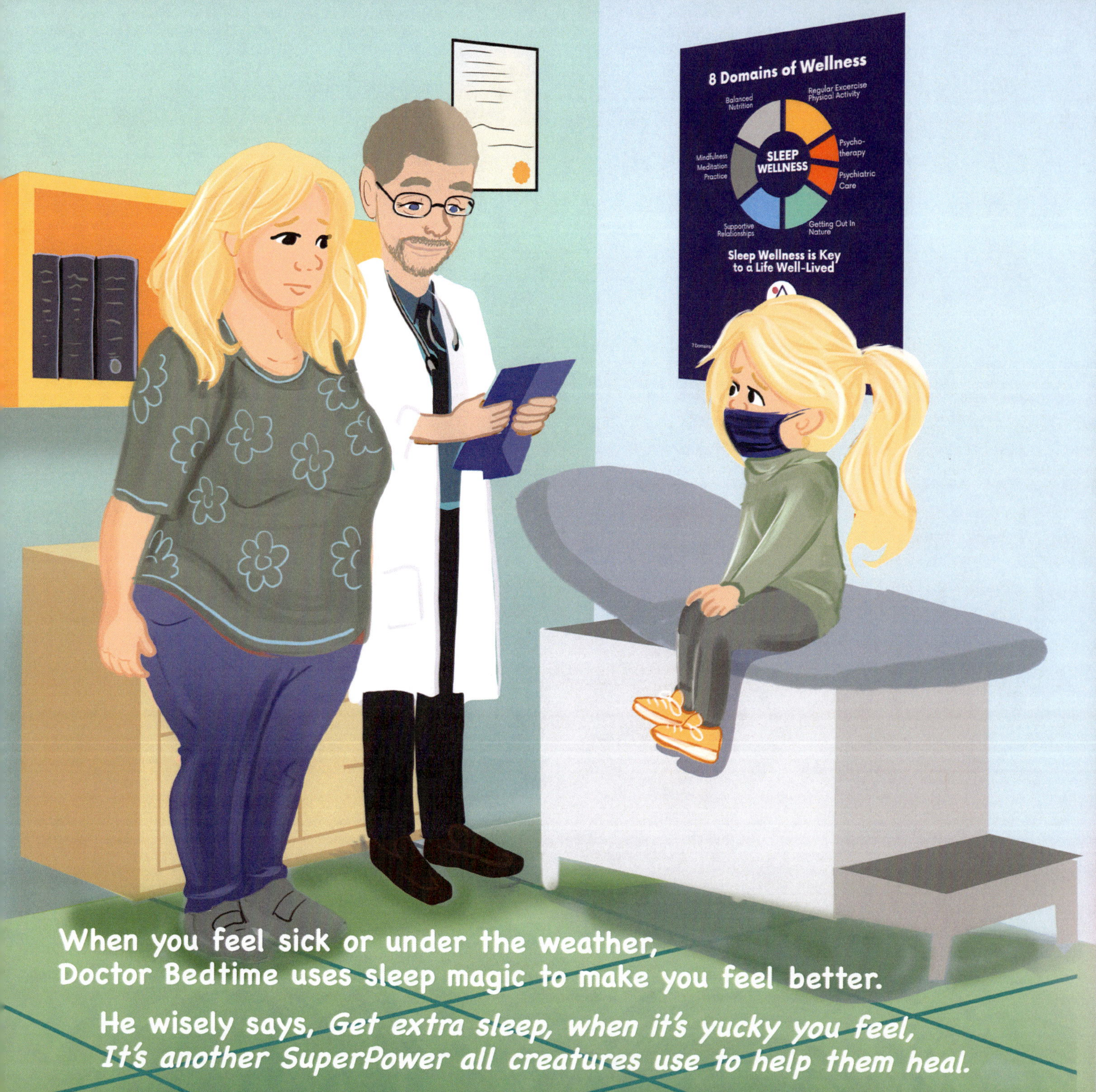

When you feel sick or under the weather,
Doctor Bedtime uses sleep magic to make you feel better.

He wisely says, *Get extra sleep, when it's yucky you feel,
It's another SuperPower all creatures use to help them heal.*

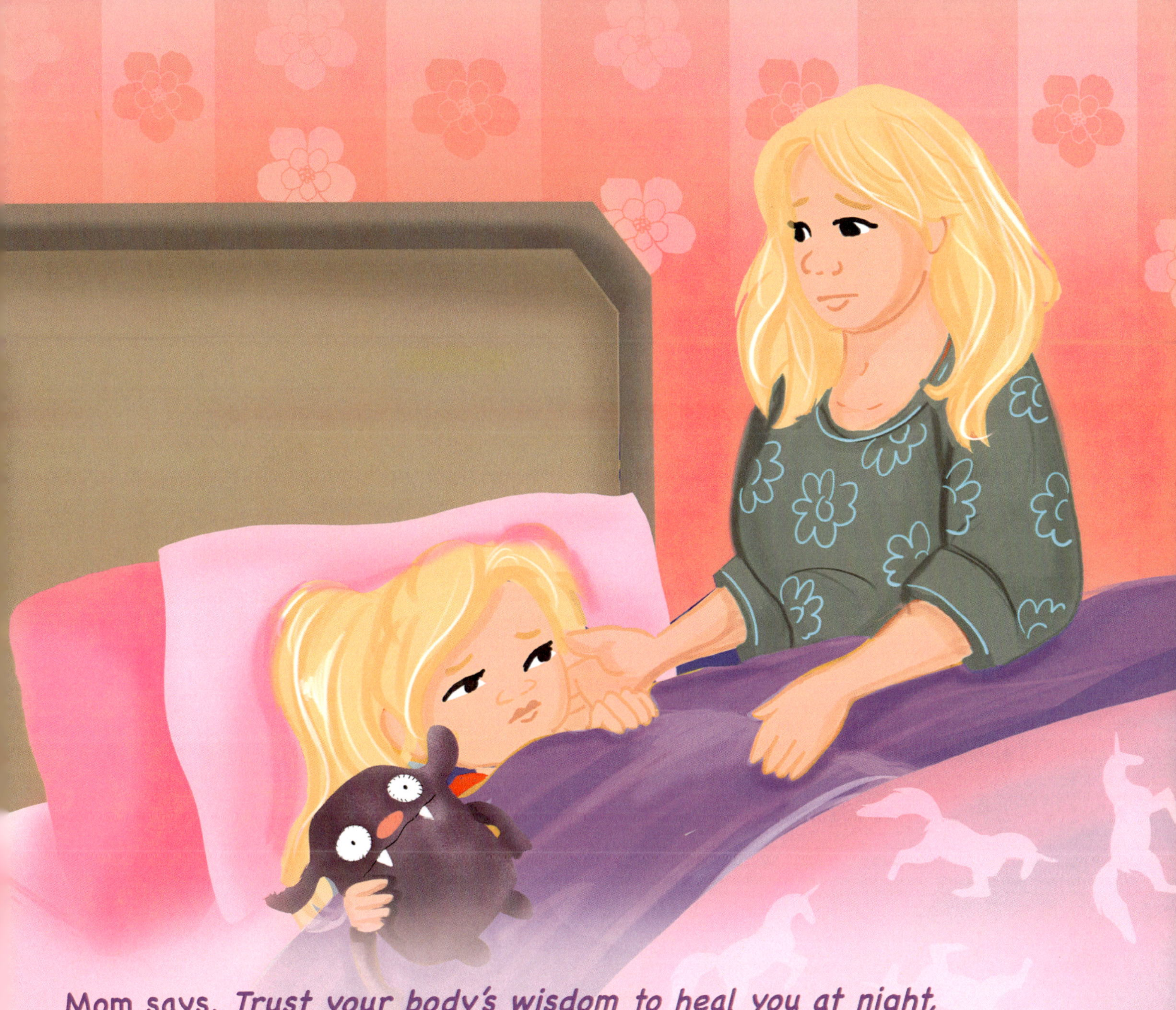

Mom says, *Trust your body's wisdom to heal you at night,*
It also knows the sleep magic it needs to feel just right.

Another reason all creatures lay down to repair and to mend,
Is for the healing comfort of sleep — it's your magical friend.

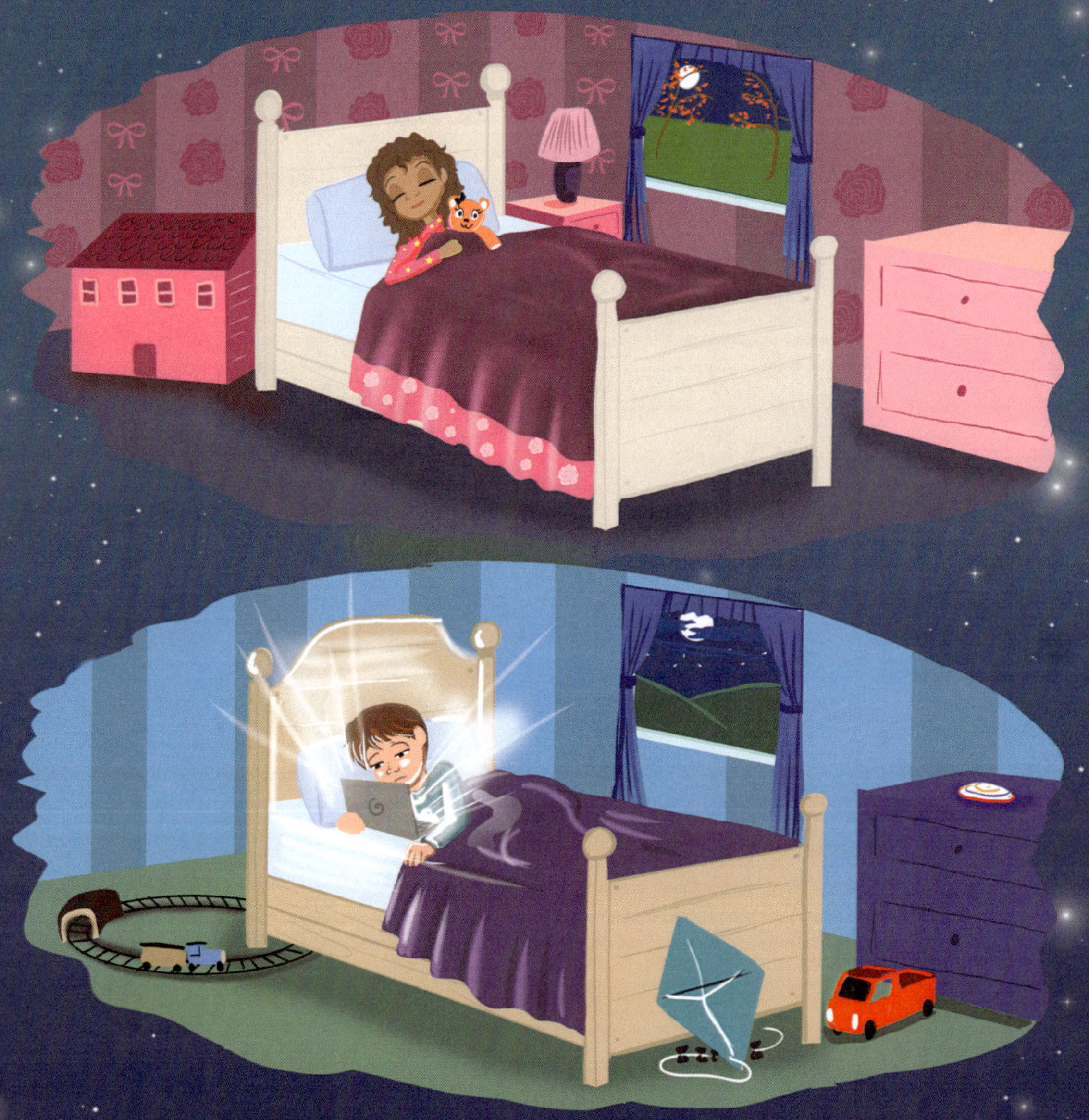

When you keep your bedtime with sleep magic to feel new,
You'll awake with SuperPower energy for all you want to do.

But, when you stay up past your bedtime to have more fun,
You'll run out of energy before the next day is done.

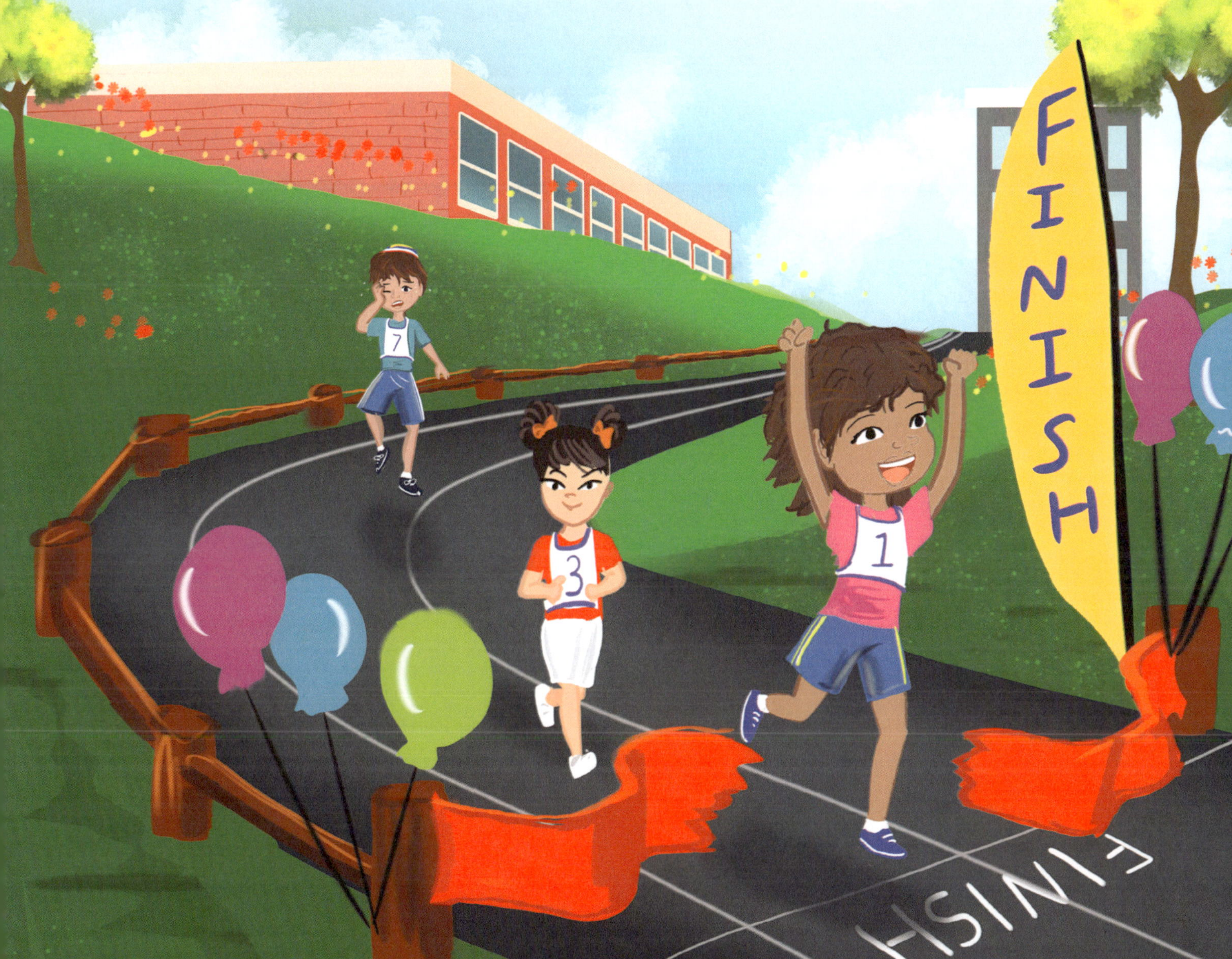

Stayed awake, did you? Got less magical sleep?
Uh, oh! You won't have enough energy when you need to compete.

So, keep your bedtime. It's your best time to energize.
You'll awake with joy, feeling new, and ready to reach for the skies!

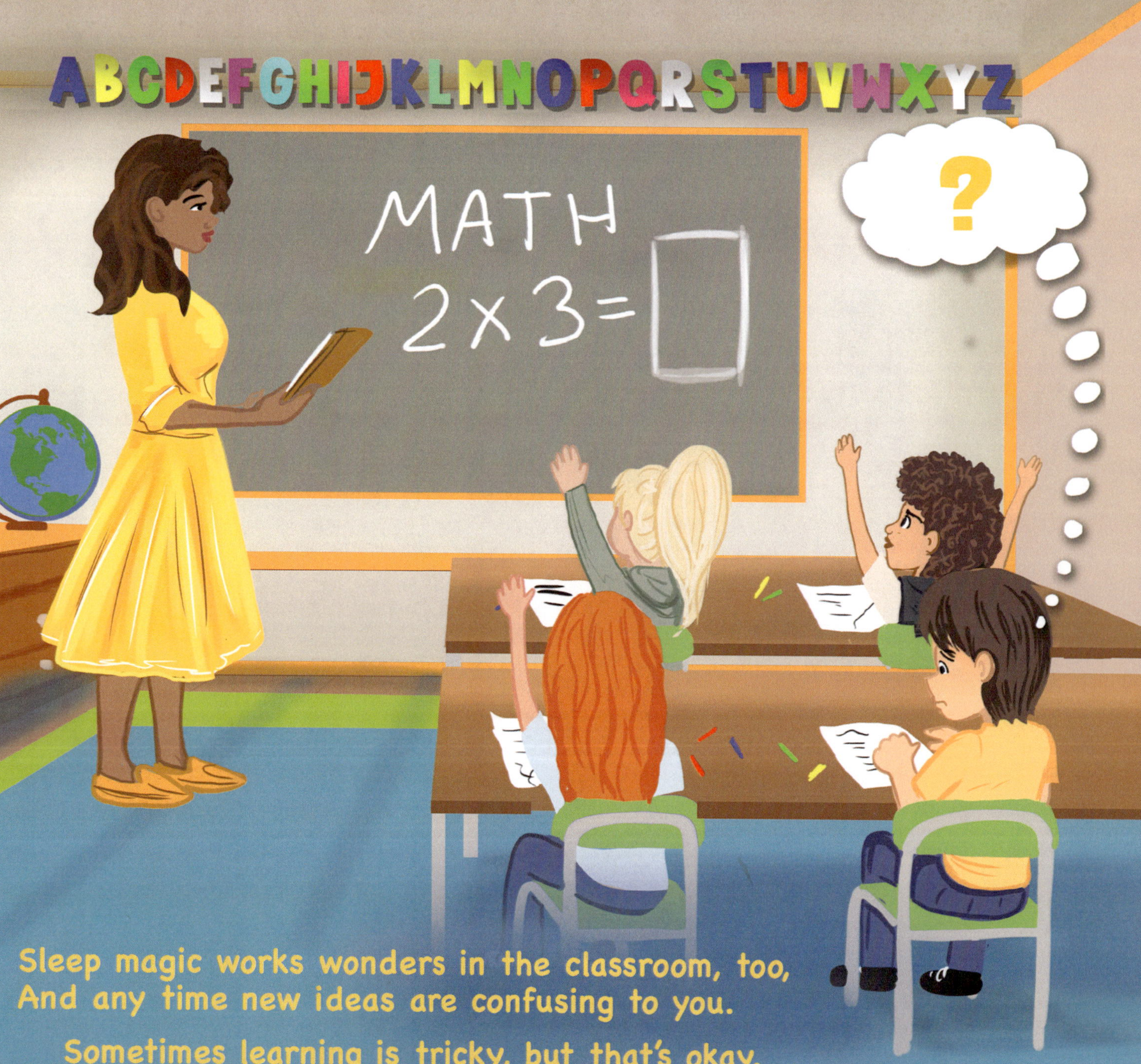

Sleep magic works wonders in the classroom, too,
And any time new ideas are confusing to you.

Sometimes learning is tricky, but that's okay.
Sleep gives you a SuperPower to learn in your unique way.

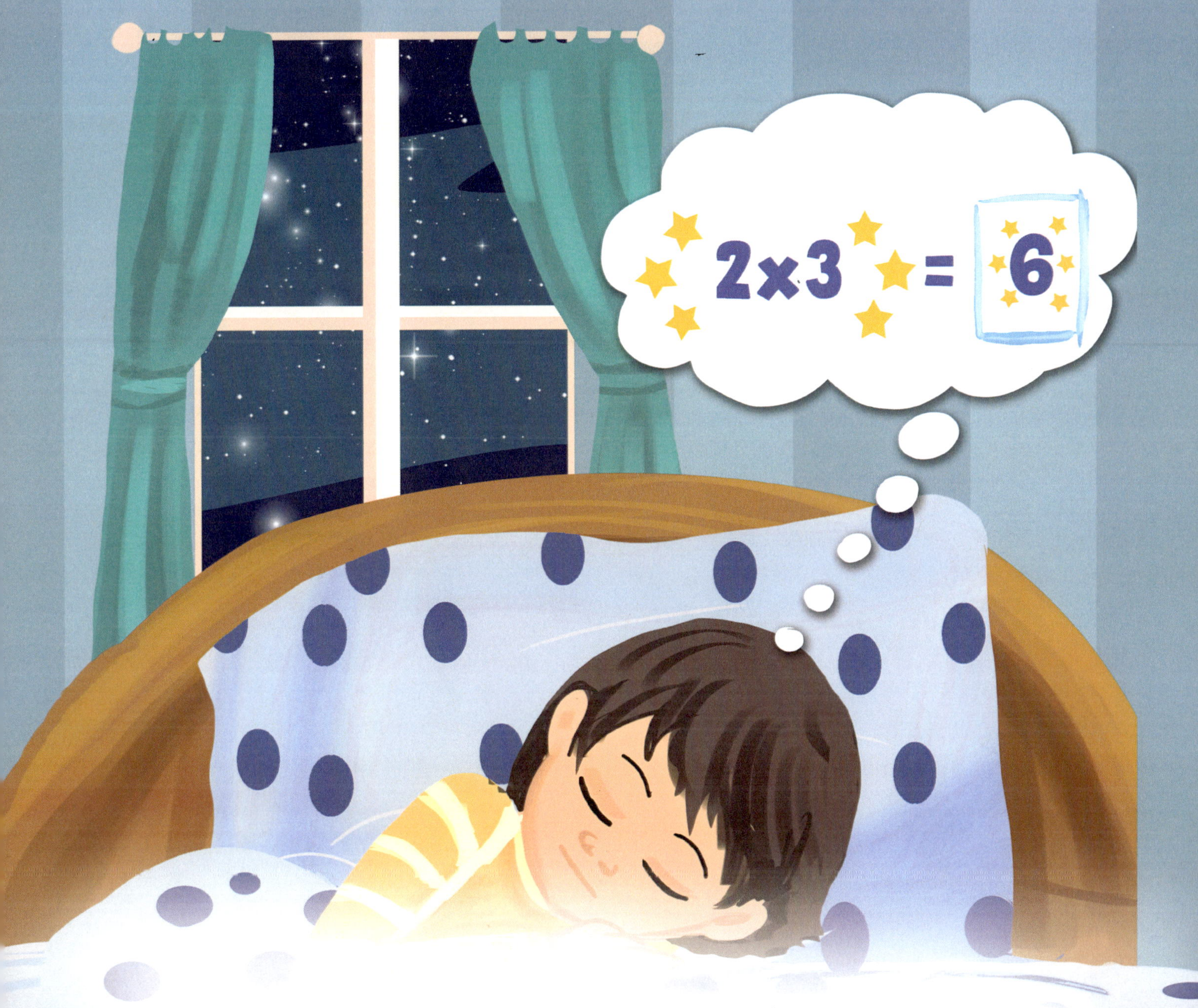

Some kids learn fast, and others take more time.
But we all need a good night's sleep to help us shine!

Sleep magic helps your brain sort, group, and review.
It's a brainy reason why we all sleep — it makes a smarter you!

When is bedtime? Same time for all creatures ending the day?
How do we know when sleep magic is on the way?

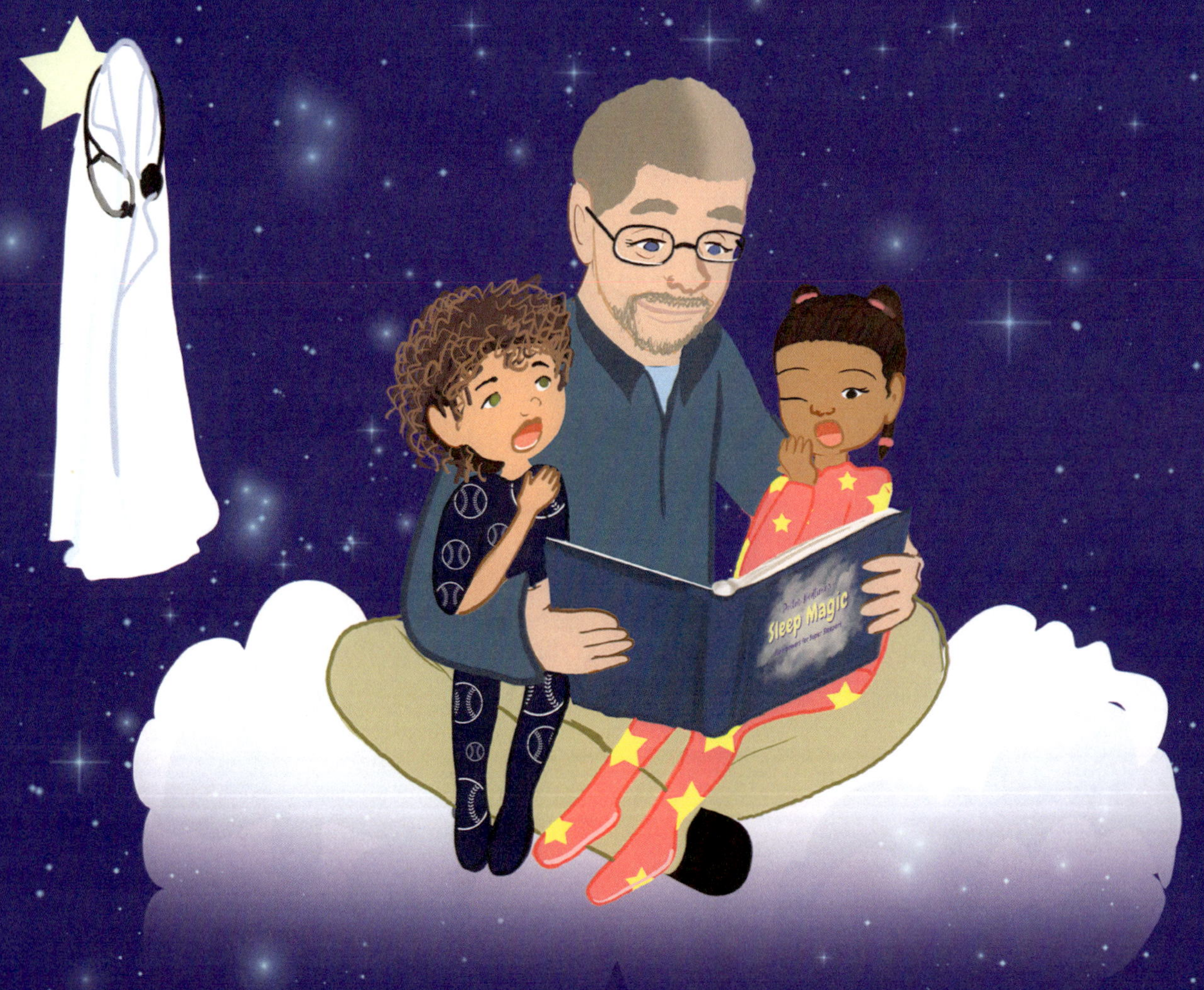

The magic of sleep can sneak up on you out of the blue!
Suddenly — you YAWN! That's often your very first clue!

Bedtime is close when other clues begin to appear,
Like rubbing your eyes, sucking your thumb, and pulling your ear.

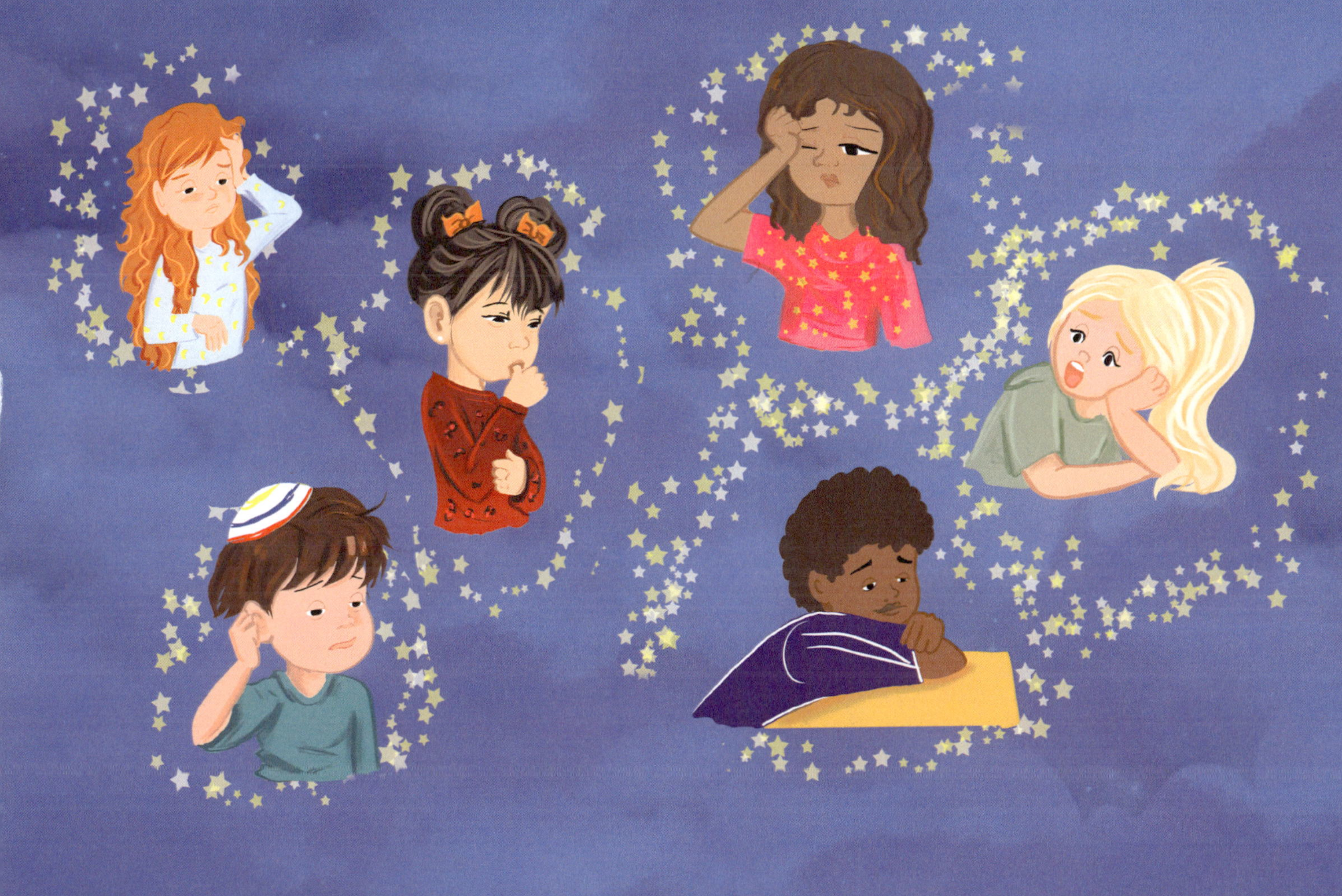

And if your head starts bobbing, it's past bedtime. Be aware!
Sleep magic is already in your safe space and waiting for you there.

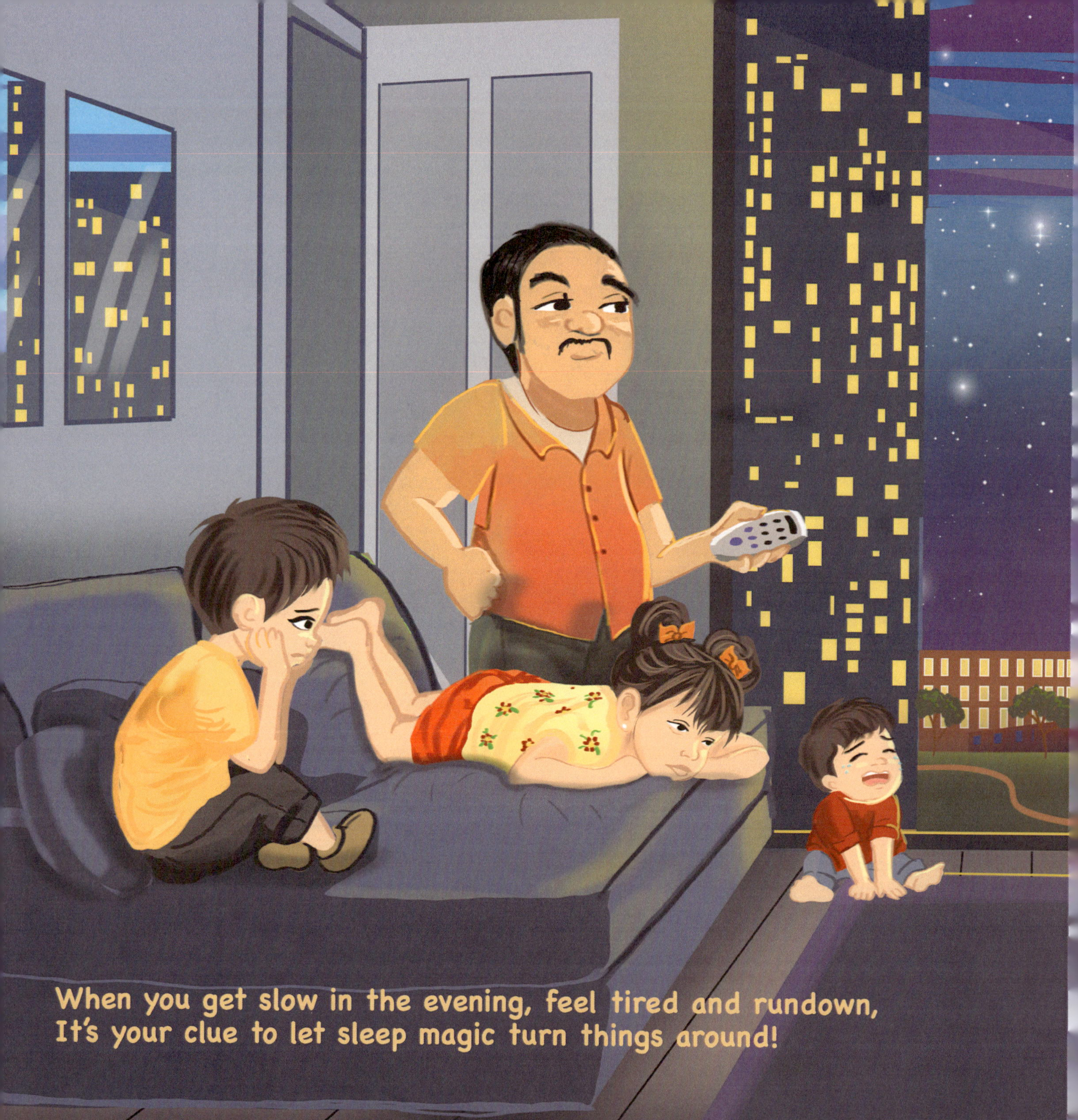
When you get slow in the evening, feel tired and rundown,
It's your clue to let sleep magic turn things around!

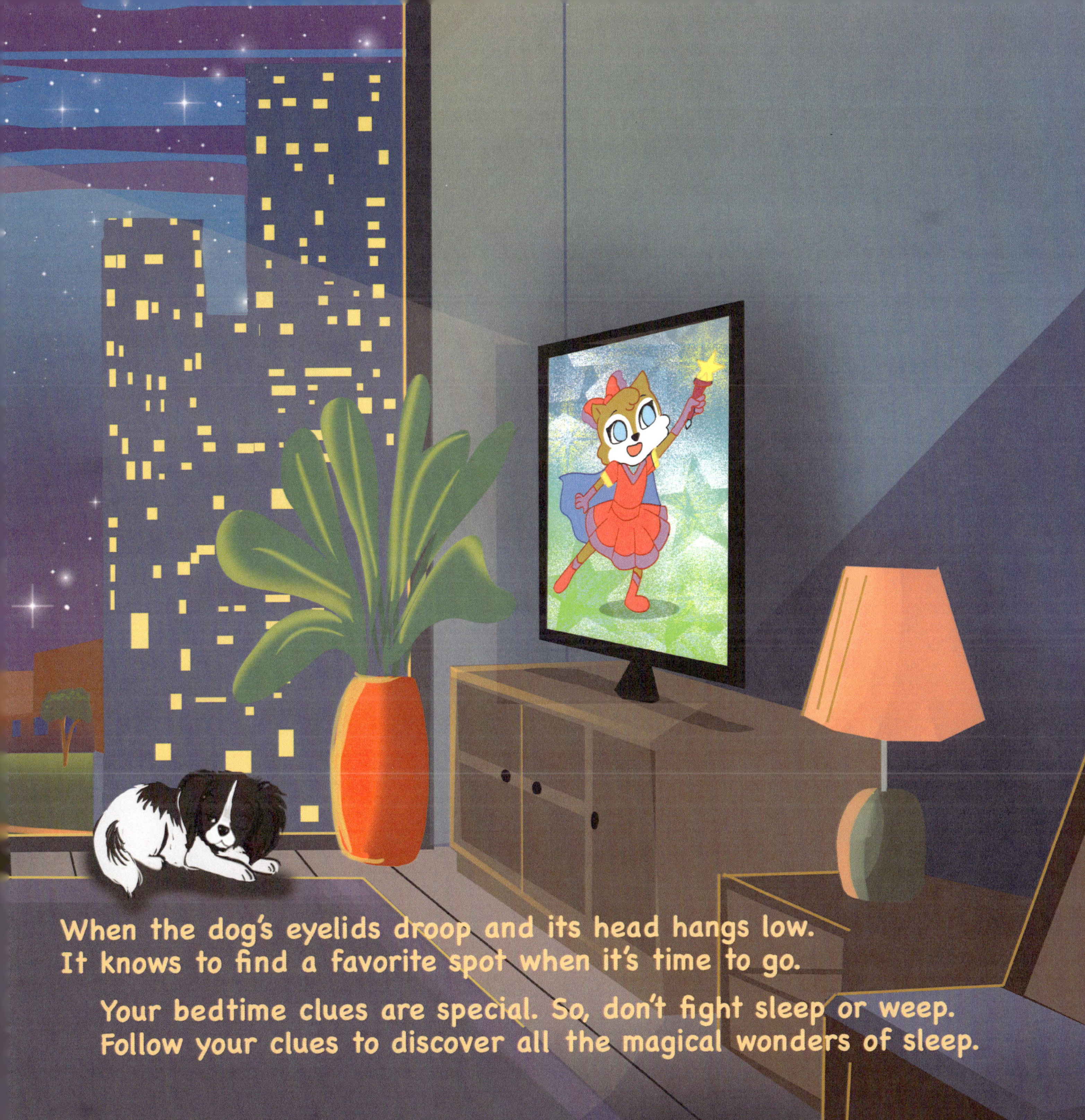

When the dog's eyelids droop and its head hangs low.
It knows to find a favorite spot when it's time to go.

Your bedtime clues are special. So, don't fight sleep or weep.
Follow your clues to discover all the magical wonders of sleep.

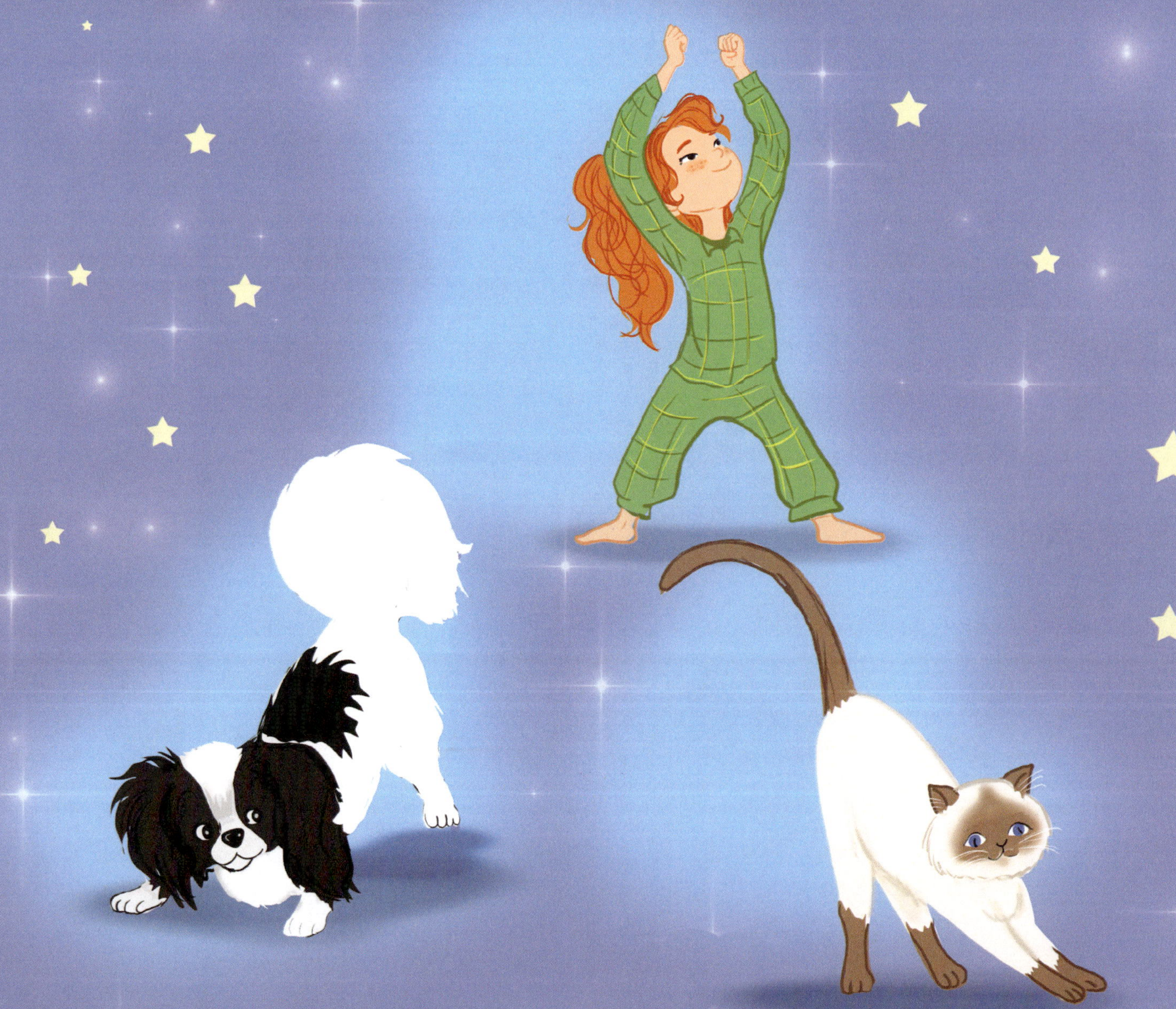

You'll know it's bedtime in another magical way,
When your body feels like stretching at the end of the day.

When you stretch like a cat or a dog, it's your clue to know
Sleep magic is coming. And it's time to go to bed and grow.

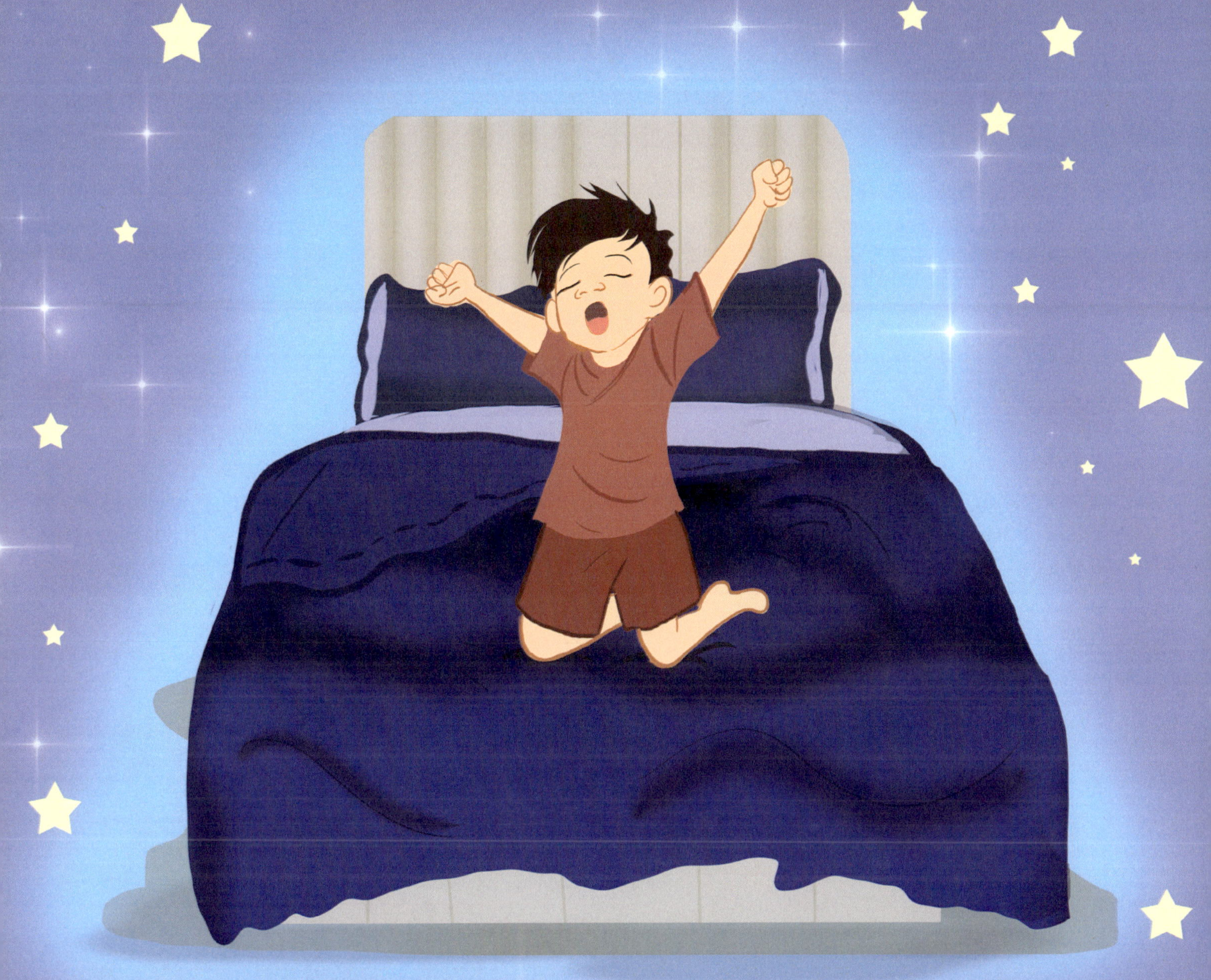

Stretch out your arms like a tall growing tree.
Reach high to the sky. Feel light and carefree.

When your muscles relax, your thoughts start to slow,
You become light as a feather, and you can let yourself go.

Dear One, now you know the sleep magic way
To grow taller, get smarter, and run faster each day.

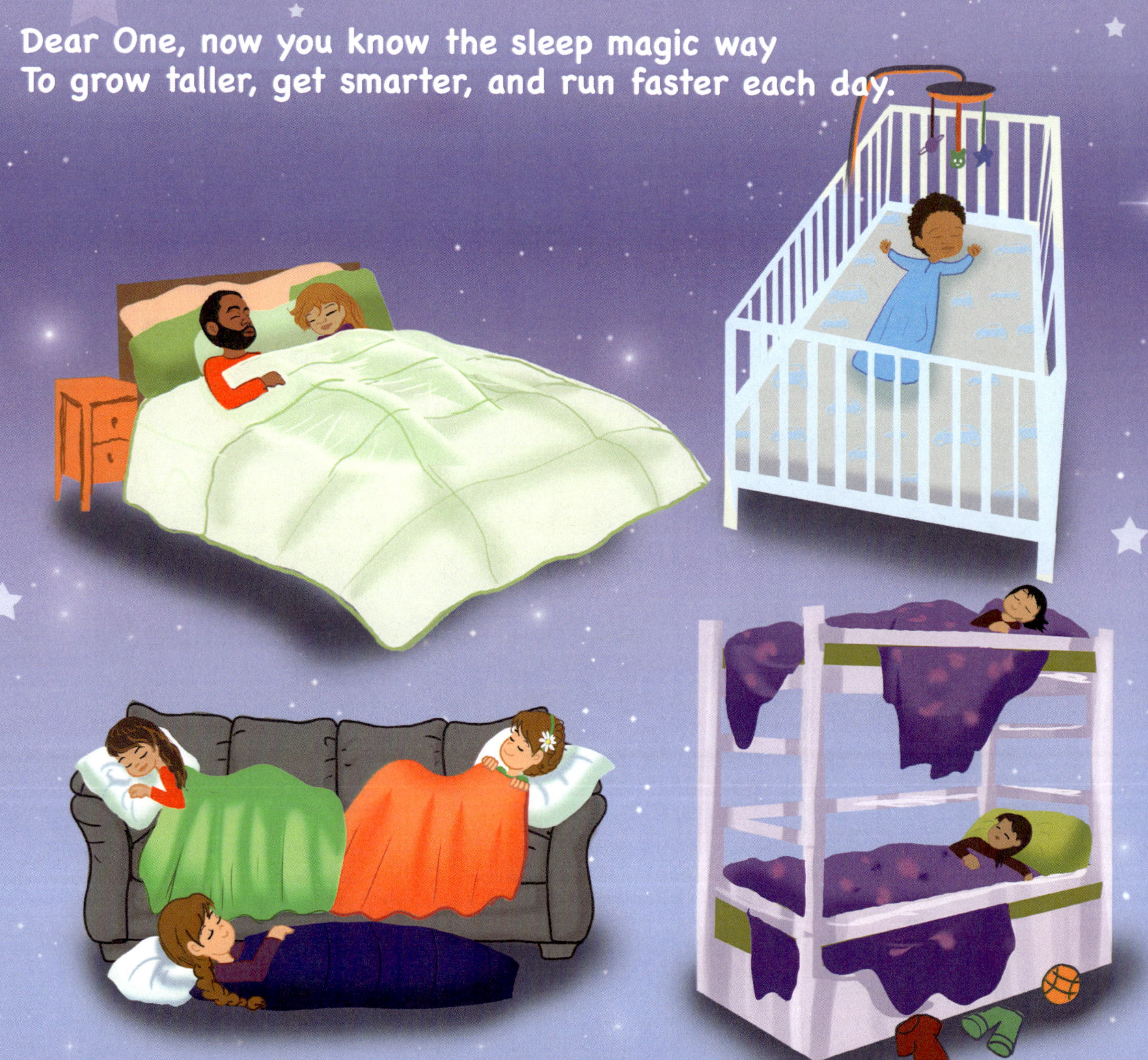

You know to snuggle up in your safe space with grateful delight,
To let your sleep magic journey begin each night.

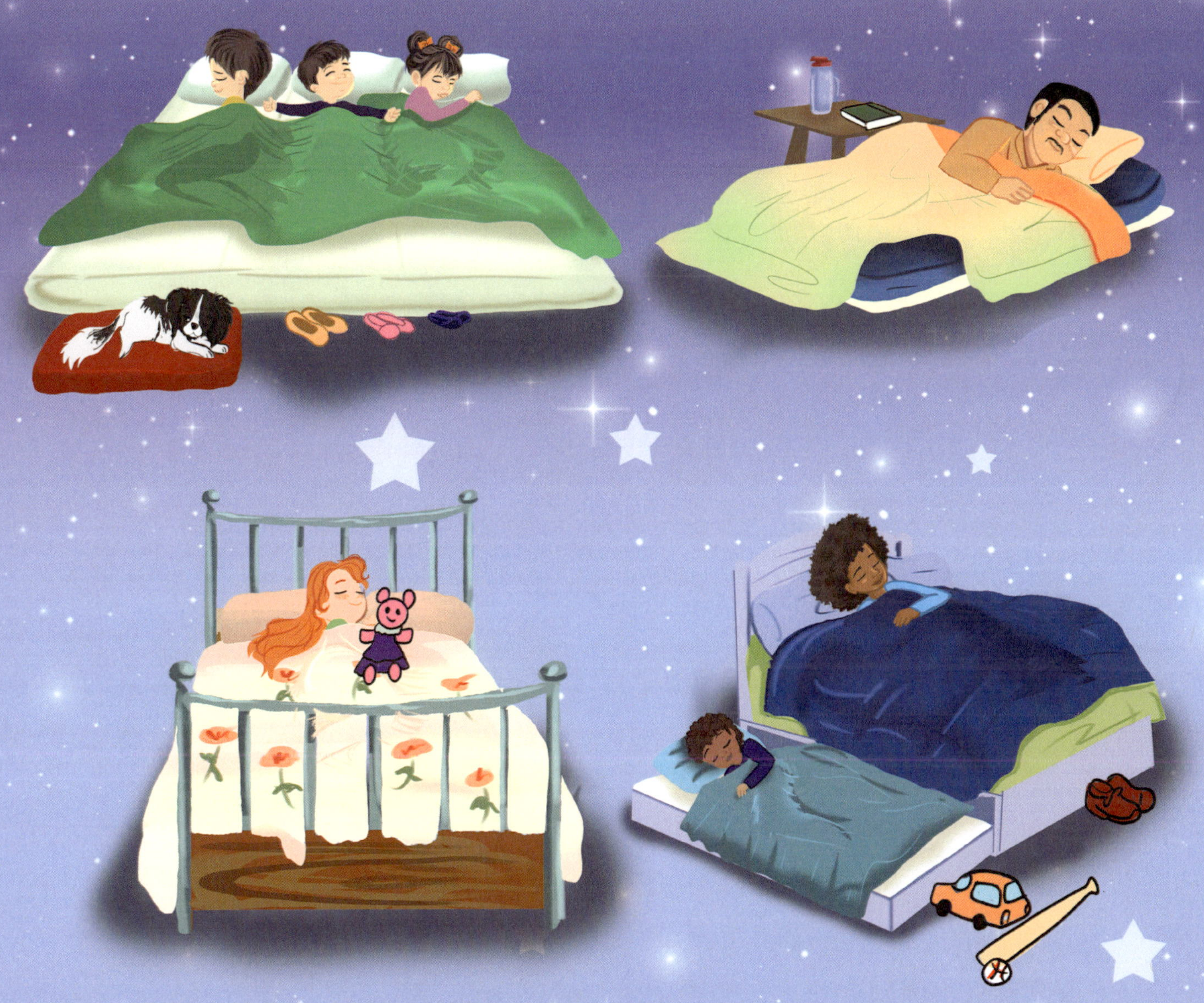

The bedtime clues you followed lead to dreams so sweet,
The dream magic begins when you drift down into sleep.

Abracadabra! Your SuperPower to dream comes alive!
Dreaming is sleep magic's most wonderful prize!

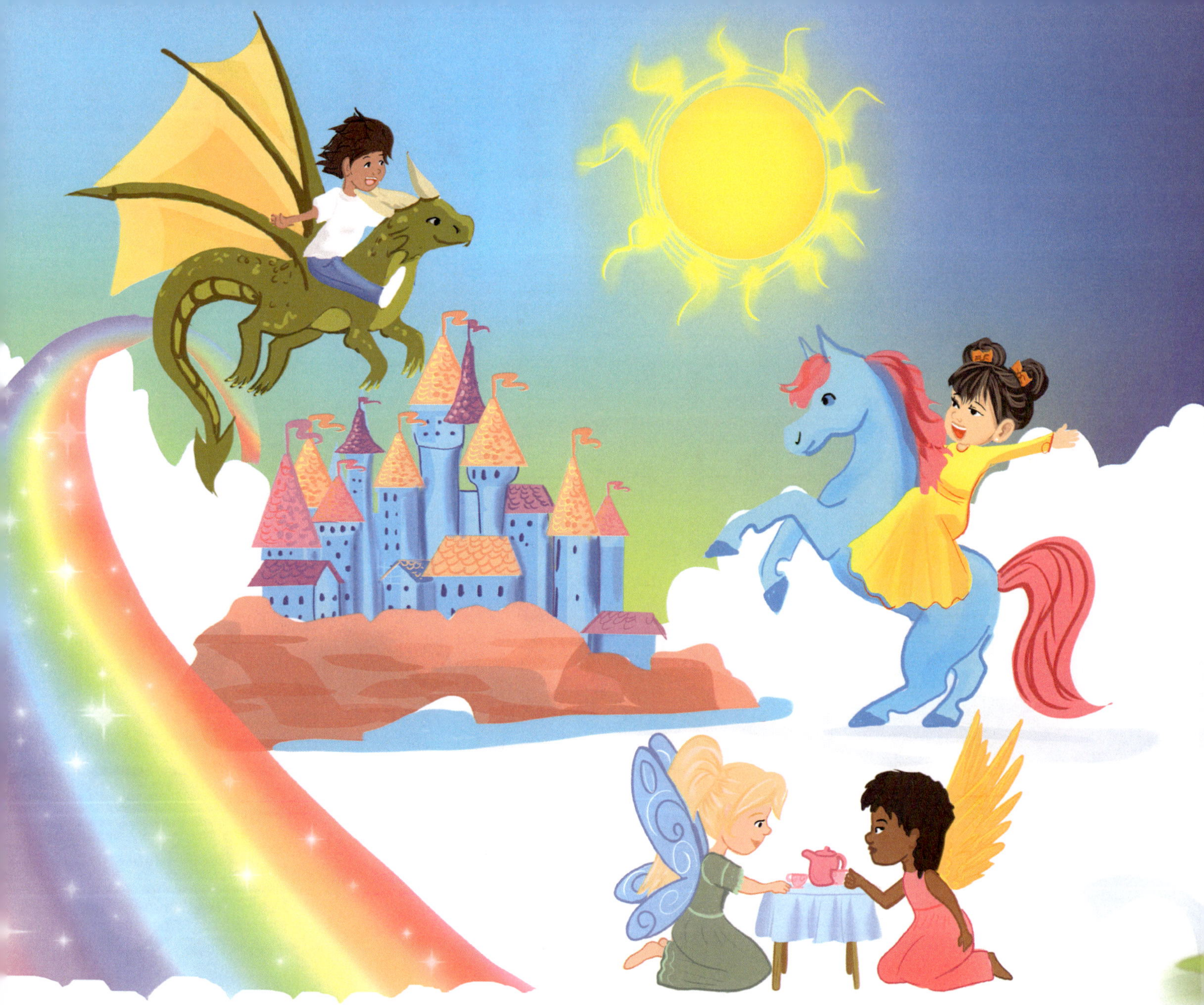

Close your eyes lightly. Let your dream SuperPower soar.
Float into new worlds with wonders to explore.

Ride green dragons and blue ponies on rainbows to castles high!
Play dress-up at tea-time. Play doctor. Kick balls to the sky.

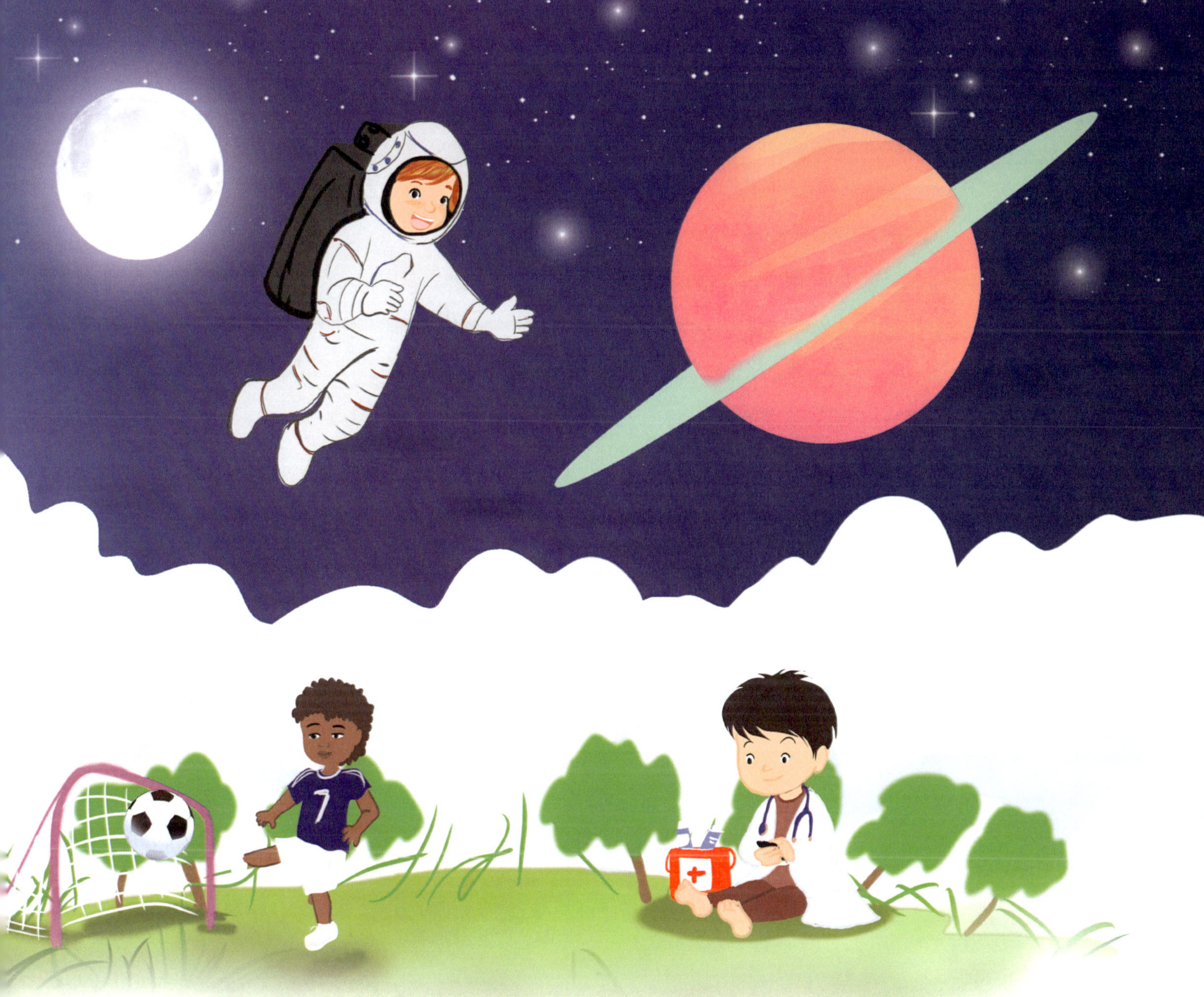

Dream magic takes you to places you wish to be;
Like an astronaut up in space, flying high, feeling free.

In dreamland, the rules are yours to make, you see,
Dreams can be as much fun as you imagine them to be.

With dream SuperPower, you can create a future too!
Planting your dream seeds will make wishes come true!

With sprinkles of sleep magic on your dream seeds each night,
Your natural gifts grow and your talents shine bright.

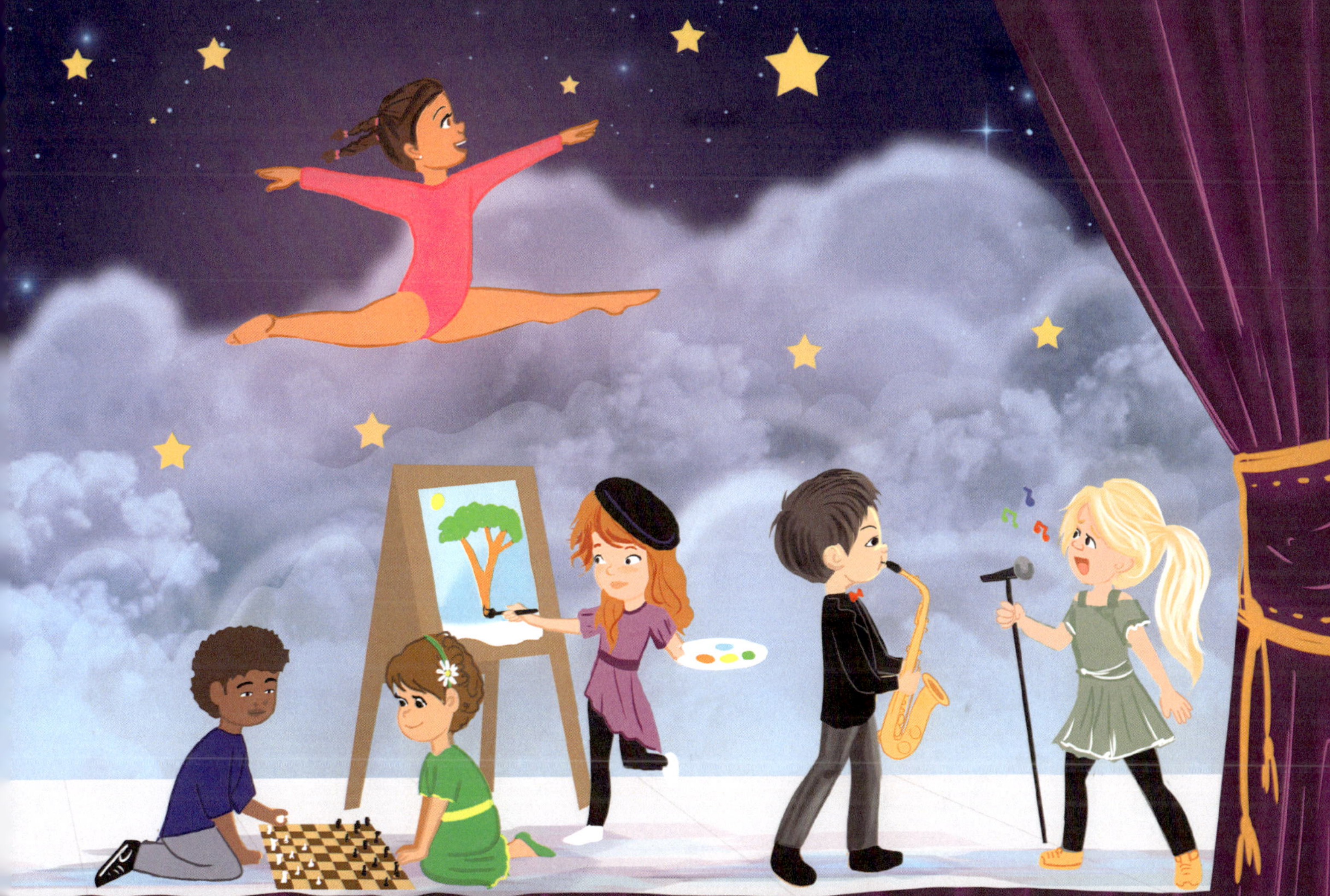

Be brave and enjoy the journey of becoming who you are.
Let sleep magic help you soar like a star.

You're a Super-Sleeper now! Always getting magical sleep you need!
Using your SuperPowers to dream big and Sleep Magic to succeed!

GOOD NIGHT AND SWEET DREAMS,
SUPER-SLEEPER!

Acknowledgments

We want to express our heartfelt appreciation to our children, Maya and Jared Washington; and Erika Clarke and Jennifer Adams, for the years of beautiful memories that brought to life many of Doctor Bedtime's Sleep Magic scenes and adventures.

We are also deeply grateful to Susan Weatherhead, Angela Devani, and Jamie Allison-Hope for their insightful and creative contributions that helped us enhance Sleep Magic's appeal to children.

Additionally, we want to acknowledge the ACEs Aware Initiative (acesaware.org) for inspiring us to prioritize children, especially those exposed to adverse childhood experiences (ACEs), in our Sleep Wellness charitable programs. The mural on the playground wall and in Doctor Bedtime's office features a poster inspired by the ACEs Aware 7 Domains of Wellness, which addresses toxic stress and trauma-related illnesses in children. The Sleep to Live Well Foundation's poster emphasizes Sleep Wellness as the 8th Domain of Wellness, highlighting its crucial role in these overall wellness practices. This poster is available for free download at www.sleeptolivewell.org

About Sleep To Live Well Foundation

The Sleep to Live Well Foundation is a 501(c)(3) private operating foundation committed to empowering individuals, especially children and their parents, along with healthcare professionals, to achieve a natural balance between quality sleep and the demands of modern life. We promote illness prevention and overall well-being through Sleep Wellness educational resources that transform sleep-resistant attitudes and habits and enhance the understanding of sleep's essential role in maintaining health and longevity.

For more information, please visit www.SleepToLiveWell.org.

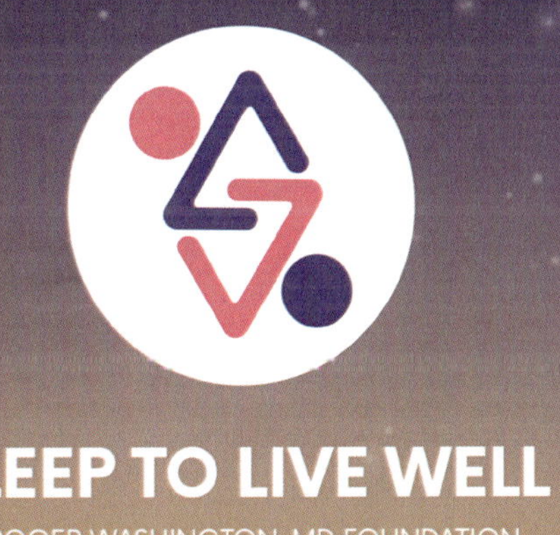

SLEEP TO LIVE WELL

A ROGER WASHINGTON, MD FOUNDATION